Dash Diet Cookbook For Beginners 2024

Transform Your Health with Flavorful and Balanced Recipes

By

BETH FROST

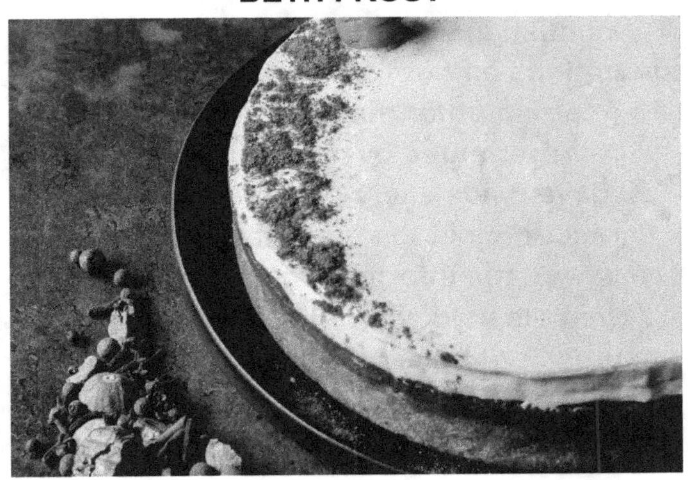

Table Of Contents

I Introduction — **10**

A. Brief overview of the DASH diet — 13

B. Importance of a healthy diet for beginners — 13

Chapter One — **14**

Understanding the DASH Diet — 14

A. Explanation of the DASH principles — 14

B. Benefits of the DASH diet for overall health — 15

C. How the DASH diet promotes cardiovascular health — 17

Chapter Two — **19**

Getting Started with the DASH Diet — 19

A. Setting realistic goals for beginners — 20

B. Grocery shopping tips and pantry essentials — 21

C. Simple meal planning strategies — 23

Chapter Three — **26**

Delicious and Nutrient-Rich Recipes — 26

A. Breakfast options promoting energy and focus — 27

B. Lunch ideas for a balanced midday meal — 29

C. Dinner recipes emphasising variety and flavour — 30

D. Snack suggestions for maintaining energy levels — 32

Chapter Four — **34**

Special Considerations and Modifications 34

A. Adapting the DASH diet for specific dietary needs 35

B. Tips for incorporating DASH principles into different lifestyles 37

C. Addressing common challenges for beginners 39

Chapter Five 42

Lifestyle Integration 42

A. Incorporating exercise into a DASH-friendly routine 44

B. Stress management and its role in a healthy lifestyle 45

C. Encouraging long-term commitment to the DASH diet 47

Chapter Six 50

Success Stories and Testimonials 50

A. Real-life experiences of individuals benefiting from the DASH diet 52

B. Before-and-after transformations 54

C. Inspirational stories to motivate beginners 56

Chapter Seven 60

Frequently Asked Questions 60

A. Addressing common queries about the DASH diet 62

B. Clarifying misconceptions and providing evidence-based answers 65

Conclusion 67

A. Recap of key DASH principles 69

B. Encouragement for beginners on their journey to better health 71

C. Final thoughts on sustaining a
DASH-friendly lifestyle.   73

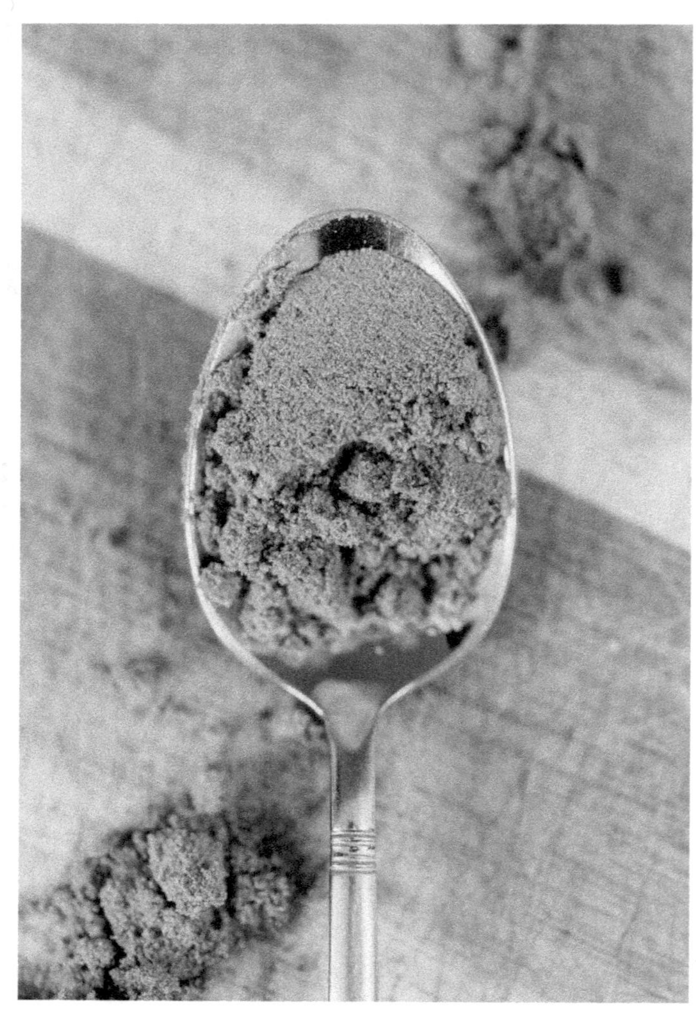

I Introduction

Embark on a journey to optimal health with the "Dash Diet Cookbook For Beginners 2024." Discover the transformative power of the Dietary Approaches to Stop Hypertension (DASH) diet, tailored specifically for those new to this wholesome approach. In this guide, we'll navigate the foundations of the DASH diet, offering practical insights, delicious recipes, and valuable tips to kickstart your path to a healthier and more vibrant lifestyle. Get ready to savor the benefits of nourishing your body with the goodness it deserves.

Welcome to "Dash Diet Cookbook for Beginners 2024: A Holistic Approach to Heart-Healthy Living." In the pages that follow, we invite you on a transformative journey towards cultivating a heart-healthy lifestyle that is both delicious and sustainable. This cookbook is more than a collection of recipes; it's a comprehensive guide designed for individuals who are ready to embrace the renowned Dietary Approaches to Stop Hypertension (DASH) principles and embark on a journey towards holistic well-being.

Understanding the Essence of DASH:
The DASH diet, initially developed to manage hypertension, has evolved into a lifestyle that transcends its origins. It's a celebration of whole,

nutrient-dense foods and a commitment to overall health. In our "Dash Diet Cookbook for Beginners 2024," we delve into the essence of the DASH principles, exploring how this approach goes beyond dietary restrictions to foster a balanced, joyful, and sustainable way of living.

A Culinary Adventure Awaits:
Embark on a culinary adventure where wholesome ingredients take center stage. Our cookbook is filled with a vibrant array of recipes, carefully crafted to not only tantalize your taste buds but also nourish your heart. From breakfast delights to satisfying main courses and delightful snacks, each recipe is a testament to the richness of flavors that can be achieved within the framework of the DASH diet.

Holistic Lifestyle Integration:
The journey towards heart-healthy living extends beyond the kitchen. That's why we've dedicated a significant portion of this cookbook to holistic lifestyle integration. Discover the art of stress management, explore practical exercise routines, and learn to foster a positive mindset. The DASH diet isn't just about what you eat; it's about creating a life that nourishes your heart in every aspect.

Navigating Meal Planning with Ease:
Meal planning is often perceived as a daunting task, but fear not. Our cookbook simplifies the process, offering practical tips and strategies to

make meal planning an enjoyable and effortless part of your routine. Create balanced, satisfying meals that align with DASH principles, promoting not only heart health but overall vitality.

Adaptable for Every Lifestyle:
We understand that everyone's journey is unique. Whether you're a vegetarian, vegan, or have specific dietary needs, our cookbook provides adaptable recipes that cater to a variety of preferences. It's about inclusivity, ensuring that the joy of heart-healthy living is accessible to all.

Real-Life Success Stories:
Interspersed throughout these pages are real-life success stories—testimonials from individuals who have experienced transformative changes through the DASH diet. Their journeys serve as inspiration, reminding us that the path to a healthier life is paved with small, consistent steps and a commitment to well-being.

Your Heart, Your Future:
As you embark on this flavorful and fulfilling journey with "Dash Diet Cookbook for Beginners 2024," remember that you hold the key to nourishing your heart and transforming your life. Every recipe, every tip, and every story shared within these pages is a step towards a healthier, happier you. Are you ready to embrace the joy of heart-healthy living? Your heart will thank you.

A. Brief overview of the DASH diet

The DASH diet, or Dietary Approaches to Stop Hypertension, is a proven eating plan designed to prevent and manage hypertension. Emphasizing whole foods, it encourages the consumption of fruits, vegetables, lean proteins, and low-fat dairy while limiting sodium intake. The DASH diet is renowned for its effectiveness in lowering blood pressure and promoting overall heart health. In this cookbook, we delve into the principles of the DASH diet, providing a concise and accessible guide for beginners to embrace this wholesome approach to nutrition.

B. Importance of a healthy diet for beginners

For beginners, adopting a healthy diet is crucial as it lays the foundation for a lifetime of well-being. A nutritious diet supports physical growth, cognitive function, and overall vitality during this formative stage. It establishes healthy eating habits that can prevent chronic illnesses, boost energy levels, and support optimal mental health. In this cookbook, we recognize the pivotal role of a healthy diet for beginners, aiming to empower individuals with the knowledge and recipes needed to kickstart a journey towards a vibrant and sustainable lifestyle.

Chapter One

Understanding the DASH Diet

The DASH diet, or Dietary Approaches to Stop Hypertension, focuses on promoting heart health and preventing hypertension. It prioritizes a balanced intake of nutrient-rich foods, emphasising fruits, vegetables, whole grains, lean proteins, and low-fat dairy. By reducing sodium consumption, the DASH diet helps lower blood pressure, reducing the risk of cardiovascular issues. In this section of the cookbook, we'll explore the core principles of the DASH diet, providing a clear grasp of its benefits and how it contributes to overall well-being.

A. Explanation of the DASH principles

1. Emphasis on Fruits and Vegetables: The DASH diet encourages a rich variety of colourful fruits and vegetables, packed with essential vitamins, minerals, and antioxidants to support overall health.

2. Whole Grains: Opting for whole grains over refined ones ensures a higher fibre content, promoting digestive health and contributing to sustained energy levels.

3. Lean Proteins: Incorporating lean protein sources, such as poultry, fish, beans, and nuts, supports muscle health and provides essential amino acids without excessive saturated fat.

4. Low-Fat Dairy: Choosing low-fat or fat-free dairy products helps maintain adequate calcium intake while minimising saturated fat content, promoting heart health.

5. Limited Sodium Intake: Reducing sodium intake is a cornerstone of the DASH diet, crucial for managing blood pressure. This involves minimising processed foods and using herbs and spices for flavouring.

6. Moderation in Sweets and Added Sugars: While not strictly eliminating sweets, the DASH diet encourages moderation in consuming sugary foods, promoting a balanced approach to nutrition.

Understanding and applying these principles form the basis of the DASH diet's effectiveness in promoting cardiovascular health and overall well-being.

B. Benefits of the DASH diet for overall health

1. Blood Pressure Management: The DASH diet is renowned for its efficacy in lowering blood pressure, reducing the risk of hypertension and related cardiovascular issues.

2. Heart Health: By promoting a balanced intake of nutrient-rich foods and minimising saturated fat, the DASH diet supports cardiovascular health, reducing the risk of heart disease.

3. Weight Management: The emphasis on whole, nutrient-dense foods aids in weight control, fostering a healthy body weight and reducing the risk of obesity-related conditions.

4. Improved Lipid Profiles: The DASH diet has been shown to positively impact lipid levels, contributing to healthier cholesterol and triglyceride levels.

5. Enhanced Nutrient Intake: The focus on fruits, vegetables, and whole grains ensures a higher intake of essential nutrients, promoting overall well-being and reducing the risk of nutritional deficiencies.

6. Diabetes Prevention: The DASH diet's emphasis on balanced, low-sodium, and low-sugar foods can contribute to better blood sugar control, reducing the risk of type 2 diabetes.

7. Reduced Inflammation: The inclusion of anti-inflammatory foods in the DASH diet can help mitigate chronic inflammation, which is linked to various health issues.

By adopting the DASH principles, individuals can experience a multitude of health benefits, contributing to a more vibrant and resilient lifestyle.

C. How the DASH diet promotes cardiovascular health

1. Blood Pressure Regulation: The DASH diet is specifically designed to lower and regulate blood pressure, reducing the risk of hypertension, a significant factor in cardiovascular issues.

2. Sodium Control: The diet's emphasis on low sodium intake helps prevent fluid retention and lower blood pressure, crucial for maintaining cardiovascular health.

3. Heart-Friendly Fats: By promoting the consumption of lean proteins and limiting saturated and trans fats, the DASH diet supports heart health and helps manage cholesterol levels.

4. Rich in Potassium, Calcium, and Magnesium: These minerals, abundant in fruits, vegetables, and low-fat dairy, play a key role in maintaining proper heart function, blood vessel dilation, and overall cardiovascular well-being.

5. Antioxidant-Rich Foods: The DASH diet encourages foods high in antioxidants, which combat oxidative stress and inflammation, contributing to a healthier cardiovascular system.

6. Weight Management: Maintaining a healthy weight through the DASH diet reduces the risk of obesity-related cardiovascular issues, such as heart disease and stroke.

7. Balanced Nutrient Profile: The diet's focus on a balanced intake of nutrients supports overall cardiovascular health, providing the body with what it needs to function optimally.

By addressing these factors, the DASH diet creates a heart-healthy eating pattern that can significantly contribute to the prevention of cardiovascular diseases and promote long-term heart well-being.

Chapter Two

Getting Started with the DASH Diet

1. Set Realistic Goals: Begin by setting achievable goals tailored to your preferences and lifestyle, making the transition to the DASH diet more manageable.

2. Educate Yourself: Familiarise yourself with the DASH principles, understanding the types of foods to emphasise and those to limit, particularly sodium-rich options.

3. Clean Out the Pantry: Rid your kitchen of high-sodium and processed foods. Stock up on whole grains, lean proteins, fruits, and vegetables to create a DASH-friendly environment.

4. Grocery Shopping Tips: Plan your grocery trips with a list focused on DASH-approved items. Choose fresh produce, lean meats, low-fat dairy, and whole grains.

5. Meal Planning Strategies: Begin with simple and balanced meal plans. Incorporate a variety of fruits and vegetables, lean proteins, and whole grains to create satisfying and nutritious meals.

6. Gradual Transition: Ease into the DASH diet by gradually introducing its principles. Start with one or two meals a day, gradually expanding to the entire day as you become more comfortable.

7. Hydration: Stay hydrated with water or other low-calorie beverages, avoiding sugary drinks. Hydration is a crucial component of the DASH diet.

By taking these steps, beginners can smoothly integrate the DASH diet into their lives, fostering a sustainable and enjoyable journey toward improved health.

A. Setting realistic goals for beginners

1. Start Gradually: Begin by incorporating DASH principles into one or two meals a day, allowing for a gradual and sustainable transition.

2. Focus on Small Changes: Instead of overhauling your entire diet, focus on making small, achievable changes, such as adding more vegetables to your meals or choosing whole grains over refined ones.

3. Understand Your Preferences: Tailor your goals to your personal tastes and preferences. Find DASH-approved foods and recipes that align with your culinary likes, making the process more enjoyable.

4. Meal Prep: Plan and prepare your meals in advance to make healthier choices easily accessible. This can prevent last-minute temptations and help you stick to your DASH goals.

5. Monitor Sodium Intake: Gradually reduce your sodium intake, starting with small adjustments. Pay attention to food labels and explore alternative ways to flavour your meals, such as using herbs and spices.

6. Celebrate Achievements: Acknowledge and celebrate your successes, no matter how small. Recognizing progress boosts motivation and reinforces the positive changes you're making.

7. Seek Support: Share your DASH journey with friends or family members. Having a support system can make the process more enjoyable and help you stay accountable to your goals.

By setting realistic and attainable goals, beginners can establish a strong foundation for long-term success with the DASH diet.

B. Grocery shopping tips and pantry essentials

1. Plan Ahead: Create a shopping list based on your planned DASH-friendly meals to avoid impulse purchases and ensure you have all necessary ingredients.

2. Shop the Perimeter: Focus on fresh produce, lean proteins, and dairy found around the perimeter of the grocery store. This minimises exposure to processed and high-sodium items in the centre aisles.

3. Read Labels: Pay attention to nutrition labels, especially sodium content. Choose products with lower sodium levels and minimal added sugars.

4. Buy Fresh Produce: Opt for a variety of colourful fruits and vegetables. Fresh produce not only adds nutritional value but also contributes to a visually appealing and diverse diet.

5. Lean Proteins: Select lean protein sources such as poultry, fish, legumes, and tofu. Aim for high-quality, unprocessed options.

6. Whole Grains: Choose whole grains like brown rice, quinoa, and whole wheat bread to increase fibre intake and promote sustained energy.

7. Low-Fat Dairy: Opt for low-fat or fat-free dairy products, such as milk and yoghourt, to maintain calcium intake while minimising saturated fat.

Pantry Essentials

1. Herbs and Spices: Build a collection of herbs and spices to flavour meals without relying on excessive salt.

2. Olive Oil: Use olive oil as a healthier alternative to saturated fats for cooking and dressings.

3. Canned Beans and Tomatoes: Keep canned beans and tomatoes on hand for quick and nutritious additions to various dishes.

4. Nuts and Seeds: Incorporate nuts and seeds for added texture, flavour, and healthy fats.

5. Whole-Grain Pasta and Rice: Stock up on whole-grain pasta and rice for versatile and fibre-rich meal options.

6. Nut Butters: Choose natural nut butters without added sugars or oils for a nutrient-dense spread.

7. Dried Herbs and Spices: Enhance flavour without added sodium by having a variety of dried herbs and spices in your pantry.

By following these tips and stocking up on these essentials, you can make your grocery trips more efficient and set yourself up for success on the DASH diet.

C. Simple meal planning strategies

1. Batch Cooking: Prepare larger quantities of DASH-approved meals and freeze individual portions for quick and convenient options throughout the week.

2. Theme Nights: Organise your meal planning around themes, such as "Meatless Monday" or "Fish Friday," making it easier to create diverse and balanced menus.

3. Build Balanced Plates: Ensure each meal includes a variety of food groups – lean proteins, whole grains, and plenty of colourful fruits and vegetables – for a balanced and satisfying plate.

4. Prep Ingredients in Advance: Wash, chop, and portion out ingredients ahead of time to streamline the cooking process during busy days.

5. Mix and Match: Create a repertoire of simple recipes and learn to mix and match ingredients to keep meals interesting while sticking to DASH principles.

6. Plan for Leftovers: Cook extra servings to have leftovers for the next day's lunch or dinner, reducing the need for frequent cooking.

7. Flexible Menus: Plan meals that allow for ingredient substitution, offering flexibility based on what's available or on sale at the grocery store.

By incorporating these strategies, meal planning becomes more manageable and sustainable, ensuring that the DASH diet aligns with your lifestyle and preferences.

Chapter Three

Delicious and Nutrient-Rich Recipes

1. Grilled Salmon with Lemon and Dill:
   - Rich in omega-3 fatty acids for heart health.
   - Served with a side of quinoa and steamed broccoli for a well-balanced meal.

2. Mango Avocado Salad:
   - Packed with vitamins and antioxidants.
   - Combines ripe mango, creamy avocado, mixed greens, and a light citrus vinaigrette.

3. Vegetarian Stir-Fry:
   - Colourful array of veggies like bell peppers, broccoli, and snap peas.
   - Tossed with tofu and a flavorful ginger-soy sauce over brown rice.

4. Turkey and Black Bean Chili:
   - Lean protein from ground turkey and fibre from black beans.
   - Seasoned with chilli spices and served with a dollop of Greek yoghourt.

5. Quinoa Stuffed Bell Peppers:
   - Quinoa, black beans, corn, and tomatoes for a protein-packed vegetarian option.

- Baked until peppers are tender and topped with a sprinkle of fresh cilantro.

6. Greek Yoghourt Parfait:
   - Layered with Greek yoghourt, fresh berries, and a sprinkle of granola.
   - Provides protein, probiotics, and a satisfying crunch.

7. Chicken and Vegetable Skewers:
   - Lean chicken breast, cherry tomatoes, and colourful bell peppers.
   - Grilled and served with a side of whole-grain couscous.

These recipes combine flavour and nutrition, showcasing the diversity and appeal of the DASH diet for beginners.

A. Breakfast options promoting energy and focus

1. Oatmeal with Berries and Almonds:
   - Whole oats for sustained energy.
   - Topped with fresh berries and almonds for antioxidants and healthy fats.

2. Greek Yoghourt Parfait:
   - Layered with Greek yoghourt, granola, and sliced bananas.

- Provides a balance of protein, fibre, and natural sugars.

3. Spinach and Feta Omelette:
   - Eggs filled with spinach, tomatoes, and feta cheese.
   - Packed with protein and essential nutrients for a hearty start.

4. Whole Grain Toast with Avocado and Poached Egg:
   - Avocado provides healthy fats, while a poached egg adds protein.
   - Whole grain toast for fibre and complex carbohydrates.

5. Smoothie Bowl with Nut Butter:
   - Blended with mixed berries, banana, and a dollop of almond butter.
   - A refreshing and nutrient-packed option.

6. Chia Seed Pudding with Mango:
   - Chia seeds soaked in almond milk topped with fresh mango.
   - Offers a dose of omega-3 fatty acids and natural sweetness.

7. Cottage Cheese and Pineapple Bowl:
   - Cottage cheese with fresh pineapple chunks.
   - High in protein and vitamin C for a light and satisfying breakfast.

These breakfast options provide a combination of macronutrients and micronutrients to fuel your day, promoting sustained energy and mental focus.

B. Lunch ideas for a balanced midday meal

1. Grilled Chicken Salad:
   - Grilled chicken breast on a bed of mixed greens.
   - Topped with cherry tomatoes, cucumber, and a light vinaigrette.

2. Quinoa and Vegetable Bowl:
   - Quinoa mixed with roasted vegetables like bell peppers, zucchini, and cherry tomatoes.
   - Drizzled with olive oil and sprinkled with feta cheese.

3. Whole Grain Wrap with Turkey and Hummus:
   - Whole grain wrap filled with lean turkey, hummus, and crisp veggies.
   - A satisfying combination of protein, fibre, and healthy fats.

4. Mediterranean Chickpea Salad:
   - Chickpeas tossed with cherry tomatoes, cucumber, red onion, and feta cheese.
   - Dressed with olive oil, lemon juice, and Mediterranean herbs.

5. Salmon and Avocado Wrap:

- Grilled salmon with avocado slices wrapped in a whole grain tortilla.
- Balanced with leafy greens and a squeeze of lime.

6. Vegetarian Quiche with Spinach and Mushrooms:
- Whole-grain crust filled with a mixture of eggs, spinach, mushrooms, and low-fat cheese.
- Baked until golden and served with a side salad.

7. Shrimp Stir-Fry with Brown Rice:
- Stir-fried shrimp with a colourful mix of broccoli, bell peppers, and snap peas.
- Served over brown rice with a soy-ginger sauce.

These lunch ideas provide a balance of proteins, carbohydrates, and vegetables, offering a satisfying and nutritious midday meal.

C. Dinner recipes emphasising variety and flavour

1. Lemon Garlic Herb Roasted Chicken:
- Whole roasted chicken marinated in a flavorful blend of lemon, garlic, and herbs.
- Served with a side of roasted vegetables for a well-rounded meal.

2. Vegetarian Stuffed Bell Peppers:
- Bell peppers filled with a mix of quinoa, black beans, corn, and spices.

- Baked until tender and topped with a zesty tomato sauce.

3. Teriyaki Salmon with Stir-Fried Vegetables:
- Salmon fillets glazed with homemade teriyaki sauce.
- Accompanied by a medley of stir-fried vegetables and brown rice.

4. Spaghetti Squash Primavera:
- Roasted spaghetti squash strands tossed with a medley of sautéed vegetables.
- Lightly seasoned with olive oil, garlic, and fresh herbs.

5. Grilled Vegetable and Chickpea Salad:
- Grilled zucchini, eggplant, and bell peppers tossed with chickpeas.
- Drizzled with balsamic vinaigrette and sprinkled with crumbled feta.

6. Turkey and Sweet Potato Chili:
- Lean ground turkey cooked with sweet potatoes, beans, and tomatoes.
- Seasoned with chilli spices for a hearty and flavorful chilli.

7. Baked Cod with Mango Salsa:
- Cod fillets baked and topped with a vibrant mango salsa.
- Served with quinoa or wild rice for a refreshing and wholesome meal.

These dinner recipes offer a diverse range of flavours and ingredients, ensuring a satisfying and enjoyable dining experience while adhering to the principles of the DASH diet.

1. Greek Yoghourt with Berries:
  - A combination of protein and antioxidants for sustained energy.

2. Almond Butter and Banana:
  - A balanced snack with healthy fats, protein, and natural sugars.

3. Hummus with Veggie Sticks:
  - Hummus paired with cucumber, carrot, and bell pepper sticks for a satisfying and nutrient-rich option.

4. Trail Mix with Nuts and Dried Fruit:
  - A mix of almonds, walnuts, and dried fruits for a portable and energising snack.

5. Whole Grain Crackers with Cheese:
  - Whole grain crackers with a slice of low-fat cheese provide a combination of carbohydrates and protein.

6. Apple Slices with Peanut Butter:

- Apple slices dipped in peanut butter for a sweet and filling snack.

7. Hard-Boiled Eggs:
- A convenient source of protein and essential nutrients to keep you energised.

8. Yogurt Parfait with Granola:
- Layered Greek yoghourt, fresh fruit, and a sprinkle of granola for a delightful and nutritious snack.

9. Edamame:
- Steamed edamame pods offer a protein-rich and satisfying snack.

10. Cottage Cheese with Pineapple:
- Cottage cheese paired with fresh pineapple chunks for a refreshing and protein-packed option.

These snacks provide a mix of macronutrients and micronutrients to help maintain energy levels between meals, supporting overall well-being.

Chapter Four

Special Considerations and Modifications

1. Gluten-Free Options:
   - Provide alternative grains like quinoa, brown rice, and gluten-free pasta for those with gluten sensitivities.

2. Vegetarian and Vegan Alternatives:
   - Include plant-based protein sources such as tofu, legumes, and tempeh to accommodate vegetarian and vegan preferences.

3. Low-Sodium Modifications:
   - Adjust recipes by reducing salt and using herbs, spices, and other flavourings to maintain taste without compromising on DASH principles.

4. Dairy-Free Substitutes:
   - Offer dairy-free alternatives like almond or coconut milk, and use plant-based spreads in recipes for those with lactose intolerance or dairy allergies.

5. Nut Allergies:
   - Provide nut-free options and alternatives such as seeds or sunflower butter for individuals with nut allergies.

6. Portion Control Guidance:

- Include tips on portion control to help individuals maintain a healthy balance, particularly for those focused on weight management.

7. Customizable Recipes:

- Encourage experimentation and customization, allowing individuals to adjust recipes based on personal preferences and dietary needs.

8. Quick and Easy Options:

- Suggest simplified versions of recipes for those with time constraints, emphasising the feasibility of incorporating DASH principles into a busy lifestyle.

Addressing these considerations ensures the adaptability of the DASH diet, making it accessible and enjoyable for individuals with diverse dietary preferences and requirements.

A. Adapting the DASH diet for specific dietary needs

1. Gluten-Free Adaptations:

- Substitute gluten-containing grains with gluten-free alternatives like quinoa, rice, or gluten-free oats.

2. Vegetarian and Vegan Modifications:

- Focus on plant-based protein sources such as legumes, tofu, and tempeh to meet protein needs for vegetarians and vegans.

3. Dairy-Free Adjustments:
- Replace dairy with non-dairy alternatives like almond milk, coconut yoghourt, or other plant-based options.

4. Low-Sodium Variations:
- Reduce sodium content by using herbs, spices, and salt-free seasonings for flavour enhancement, and choose low-sodium or no-salt-added ingredients.

5. Nut-Free Alternatives:
- Offer seeds, seed butters, or other non-nut alternatives for those with nut allergies.

6. Customizable Recipes:
- Provide a variety of ingredient options within recipes, allowing individuals to tailor meals to their dietary preferences and restrictions.

7. Balancing Macronutrients:
- Adjust macronutrient ratios to accommodate specific dietary needs, such as increasing healthy fats for those on a higher-fat diet.

8. Individualised Portion Guidance:

- Offer guidance on portion sizes to meet the nutritional needs of individuals with varying calorie requirements.

By incorporating these adaptations, the DASH diet can be tailored to address specific dietary needs while maintaining its core principles of promoting heart health and overall well-being.

B. Tips for incorporating DASH principles into different lifestyles

1. Busy Professionals:
- Opt for quick and easy DASH-approved recipes that require minimal preparation.
- Batch cook meals on weekends for convenient grab-and-go options during the week.

2. Families with Children:
- Make DASH-friendly meals appealing to children by incorporating colourful fruits and vegetables in creative ways.
- Involve kids in meal planning and preparation to encourage a positive relationship with nutritious foods.

3. Vegetarians and Vegans:
- Focus on plant-based protein sources like legumes, tofu, and nuts to meet protein needs.
- Experiment with diverse vegetarian and vegan recipes to keep meals exciting and satisfying.

4. Fitness Enthusiasts:

   - Choose recipes that align with increased energy demands, incorporating lean proteins and complex carbohydrates.

   - Emphasise hydration with water and include electrolyte-rich foods like fruits and vegetables.

5. Seniors:

   - Adapt recipes to suit individual dietary preferences and any specific nutritional requirements.

   - Consider smaller, more frequent meals to accommodate appetite changes.

6. College Students:

   - Opt for budget-friendly recipes that are easy to prepare with limited kitchen equipment.

   - Utilise meal prep to save time and ensure access to nutritious options during busy study periods.

7. Travellers:

   - Pack DASH-friendly snacks like nuts, seeds, and dried fruits for on-the-go nutrition.

   - Choose restaurants that offer whole food options and prioritise grilled or steamed dishes.

8. Social Gatherings:

   - Plan and bring DASH-approved dishes to social events to ensure there are healthy options available.

- Communicate dietary preferences to hosts to facilitate a supportive and inclusive environment.

By tailoring DASH principles to different lifestyles, individuals can seamlessly integrate this heart-healthy approach into their daily routines, promoting sustainable and enjoyable adherence to the diet.

C. Addressing common challenges for beginners

1. Meal Planning Overwhelm:
  - Start with simple and familiar recipes, gradually incorporating new ones.
  - Plan meals for the week ahead to reduce decision-making stress.

2. Sodium Reduction Difficulties:
  - Gradually decrease salt in recipes to allow taste buds to adjust.
  - Use herbs, spices, and other flavourings to enhance taste without relying on salt.

3. Incorporating More Vegetables:
  - Experiment with different cooking methods to find what makes vegetables more appealing.
  - Sneak veggies into favourite dishes, like adding spinach to pasta sauce or blending them into smoothies.

4. Balancing Macronutrients:

- Focus on balanced meals with a mix of protein, carbohydrates, and healthy fats.
- Use tools like food tracking apps initially to develop an understanding of portion sizes.

5. Time Constraints:

- Prioritise simple and quick recipes, emphasising batch cooking for efficiency.
- Pre-cut and prep ingredients in advance to streamline the cooking process.

6. Social Situations:

- Communicate dietary preferences to friends and family to ensure supportive environments during gatherings.
- Offer to bring a DASH-friendly dish to social events to guarantee a nutritious option.

7. Cravings for Processed Foods:

- Gradually reduce processed foods, replacing them with whole food alternatives.
- Allow occasional treats to avoid feelings of deprivation.

8. Limited Culinary Skills:

- Start with beginner-friendly recipes and gradually expand cooking skills.
- Utilise online resources, cooking classes, or cookbooks for guidance and inspiration.

By acknowledging and addressing these common challenges, beginners can navigate the initial stages of adopting the DASH diet more effectively, setting the stage for long-term success in maintaining a heart-healthy lifestyle.

Chapter Five

Lifestyle Integration

1. Exercise Routine:
   - Pair the DASH diet with regular physical activity for comprehensive cardiovascular health.
   - Choose activities you enjoy to make exercise a sustainable part of your lifestyle.

2. Stress Management:
   - Incorporate stress-reducing activities such as mindfulness, meditation, or yoga.
   - Prioritize self-care to maintain emotional well-being alongside a healthy diet.

3. Hydration Habits:
   - Ensure adequate water intake throughout the day to support overall health and hydration.
   - Incorporate herbal teas or infused water for variety and added flavor.

4. Mealtime Environment:
   - Create a pleasant dining environment, focusing on mindful eating without distractions.
   - Share meals with loved ones to enhance the social aspect of dining.

5. Quality Sleep:

- Establish a consistent sleep routine for better overall health.
   - Avoid heavy meals close to bedtime to promote restful sleep.

6. Social Connections:
   - Share DASH-friendly meals with friends and family to foster social connections.
   - Encourage loved ones to join you in adopting a heart-healthy lifestyle.

7. Flexibility and Enjoyment:
   - Embrace flexibility in your approach, recognizing that occasional indulgences can coexist with a healthy lifestyle.
   - Experiment with new recipes and flavors to keep the diet enjoyable.

8. Long-Term Commitment:
   - View the DASH diet as a sustainable, long-term commitment rather than a short-term solution.
   - Celebrate milestones and positive changes to stay motivated on your health journey.

By integrating the DASH diet into various aspects of your lifestyle, you can create a holistic approach to well-being that promotes not only heart health but also overall physical and mental wellness.

1. Choose Enjoyable Activities:
- Engage in exercises you enjoy, whether it's walking, cycling, swimming, or dancing, to make physical activity a positive part of your routine.

2. Pair Workouts with Meals:
- Schedule workouts around meal times to establish a consistent routine.
- A post-meal walk can aid digestion and contribute to overall well-being.

3. Create a Home Workout Space:
- Set up a dedicated space at home for quick and convenient workouts, reducing barriers to exercise.
- Include simple equipment like resistance bands or dumbbells for added variety.

4. Join Group Classes or Clubs:
- Participate in group fitness classes or sports clubs to make exercise social and enjoyable.
- Team up with friends or family for shared activities, fostering a supportive environment.

5. Incorporate Interval Training:
- Include high-intensity interval training (HIIT) or short bursts of intense exercise to maximize efficiency and burn calories.

6. Combine Cardio and Strength Training:

- Integrate both cardiovascular exercises (e.g., jogging, cycling) and strength training to enhance overall fitness.
- Aim for a well-rounded routine that includes flexibility and balance exercises.

7. Set Realistic Goals:

- Establish achievable exercise goals that align with your fitness level and schedule.
- Gradually increase intensity and duration to progress over time.

8. Prioritize Consistency:

- Focus on consistent, regular exercise rather than sporadic intense workouts.
- Aim for at least 150 minutes of moderate-intensity aerobic activity per week, as recommended by health guidelines.

By blending DASH-friendly eating habits with a consistent and enjoyable exercise routine, you can create a comprehensive approach to promoting cardiovascular health and overall well-being.

B. Stress management and its role in a healthy lifestyle

1. Impact on Physical Health:

- Chronic stress can contribute to various health issues, including cardiovascular problems, compromised immune function, and digestive issues.

2. Mental Well-Being:
- Effective stress management supports mental health, reducing the risk of anxiety, depression, and other mental health disorders.

3. Healthy Coping Mechanisms:
- Develop and incorporate healthy coping mechanisms such as mindfulness, meditation, deep breathing exercises, or engaging in hobbies to reduce stress levels.

4. Improved Sleep:
- Stress management contributes to better sleep quality, which is essential for overall well-being and maintaining energy levels.

5. Enhanced Resilience:
- Building stress resilience helps individuals navigate challenges with a more positive mindset, preventing the negative impact of stress on health.

6. Positive Impact on Eating Habits:
- Managing stress reduces the likelihood of emotional eating or turning to unhealthy comfort foods, supporting a balanced and nutritious diet.

7. Regular Physical Activity:
- Exercise is a powerful stress-reliever, releasing endorphins and promoting a sense of well-being.

- Incorporate regular physical activity into your routine for holistic stress management.

8. Social Connections:
  - Maintaining strong social connections provides emotional support during stressful times.
  - Share experiences with friends or family, fostering a sense of community and understanding.

9. Time Management:
  - Effective time management reduces stress related to deadlines and pressures.
  - Prioritize tasks, delegate when possible, and set realistic goals to create a sense of control.

10. Mindful Eating:
  - Practice mindful eating by being present during meals, savoring each bite, and paying attention to hunger and fullness cues.

By actively incorporating stress management techniques into your daily life, you can create a foundation for a healthier and more balanced lifestyle, promoting both physical and mental well-being.

C. Encouraging long-term commitment to the DASH diet

1. Educate on Health Benefits:

- Emphasize the long-term health benefits of the DASH diet, including improved heart health, reduced hypertension, and overall well-being.

2. Gradual Integration:

- Encourage a gradual and sustainable approach to adopting the DASH diet, allowing individuals to make lasting lifestyle changes.

3. Personalization:

- Emphasize the flexibility of the DASH diet, allowing individuals to tailor it to their preferences and dietary needs for a more personalized and enjoyable experience.

4. Small Celebrations:

- Acknowledge and celebrate small victories along the way, reinforcing the positive changes individuals make in their eating habits.

5. Social Support:

- Foster a supportive community by connecting individuals with similar health goals, either in person or through online platforms, providing encouragement and accountability.

6. Regular Check-Ins:

- Schedule regular check-ins to assess progress, address challenges, and make adjustments to the DASH diet plan as needed.

7. Mindful Eating Practices:

- Encourage mindful eating habits, promoting awareness of hunger and fullness cues, and savoring the flavors of DASH-friendly meals.

8. Educational Resources:
- Provide ongoing access to educational resources, recipes, and tips to keep individuals engaged and informed about the principles and benefits of the DASH diet.

9. Variety in Meals:
- Emphasize the diversity of foods within the DASH diet, showcasing the richness of flavors and ingredients to keep meals interesting over the long term.

10. Integration with Lifestyle:
- Integrate DASH principles into various aspects of daily life, including social events, holidays, and travel, ensuring its compatibility with different situations.

By fostering a positive and adaptable approach, individuals are more likely to sustain their commitment to the DASH diet as a long-term lifestyle choice, promoting enduring health benefits.

Chapter Six

Success Stories and Testimonials

1. Heart Health Improvement:
   - "After adopting the DASH diet, my blood pressure significantly decreased, and my doctor was impressed with the positive changes in my heart health. It's a sustainable lifestyle that I'm proud to maintain."

2. Weight Loss Journey:
   - "The DASH diet not only helped me manage my blood pressure but also supported my weight loss goals. The variety of delicious meals made the journey enjoyable, and I feel healthier and more energetic than ever."

3. Family Well-Being:
   - "As a family, we decided to embrace the DASH diet together. Not only have we seen improvements in our health, but it has also become a bonding experience. Cooking and enjoying nutritious meals together is now a cherished part of our daily routine."

4. Increased Energy and Focus:
   - "Since integrating the DASH principles into my lifestyle, I've noticed a significant boost in energy

and focus. It's amazing how the right food choices can positively impact every aspect of your life."

5. Lifestyle Transformation:
   - "The DASH diet has been a game-changer for me. It's not just about what I eat; it's a holistic approach to health. From stress management to regular exercise, the DASH lifestyle has transformed my overall well-being."

6. Culinary Exploration:
   - "Embarking on the DASH diet introduced me to a world of delicious and nutritious recipes. I never knew healthy eating could be so flavorful. It's not a diet; it's a culinary adventure."

7. Supportive Community:
   - "Being part of a community that shares the DASH journey has been instrumental in my success. The support, recipe ideas, and shared experiences make it feel like we're all in this together."

8. Maintaining Balance:
   - "The DASH diet has taught me the importance of balance in my meals and in life. I no longer view it as a restrictive diet but as a sustainable way of living that brings harmony to my health."

These testimonials showcase the positive impact of the DASH diet on various aspects of individuals' lives, from heart health and weight management to overall well-being and a sense of community.

A. Real-life experiences of individuals benefiting from the DASH diet

1. John's Blood Pressure Success:
   - "After being diagnosed with hypertension, I decided to try the DASH diet. Within a few months, my blood pressure readings normalized. It's incredible how simple changes in eating habits can have such a profound impact."

2. Emily's Weight Loss Journey:
   - "I struggled with weight for years. The DASH diet became my guiding light. Not only did it help me shed pounds, but it also taught me to appreciate wholesome foods. It's not a diet; it's a sustainable lifestyle."

3. Sarah's Family Transformation:
   - "As a mom, I wanted to instill healthy eating habits in my family. The DASH diet allowed us to embrace nutritious meals together. Now, my kids actually enjoy vegetables, and we've all experienced positive health changes."

4. Mike's Energy Boost:
   - "I was always feeling sluggish, and my diet was full of processed foods. Switching to the DASH diet

was a game-changer. My energy levels soared, and I no longer rely on sugary snacks for a pick-me-up."

5. Linda's Culinary Discovery:
   - "I thought healthy eating meant bland meals, but the DASH diet proved me wrong. Exploring new recipes with fresh ingredients has become a joy. Who knew eating well could be so delicious?"

6. Chris' Stress Reduction:
   - "Stress used to be a constant companion. Incorporating DASH principles not only improved my blood pressure but also taught me valuable stress management techniques. It's about holistic well-being."

7. Jenna's Supportive Community:
   - "Joining DASH diet communities online connected me with like-minded individuals. We share recipes, tips, and encouragement. It's more than a diet; it's a supportive network that keeps me motivated."

8. Tom's Heart-Healthy Lifestyle:
   - "Heart disease runs in my family, so I turned to the DASH diet for preventive measures. It's now a lifestyle that ensures my heart stays healthy. My doctor is impressed with the positive changes in my overall cardiovascular health."

These real-life experiences highlight the diverse ways in which individuals have benefited from adopting the DASH diet, whether through improved health markers, weight loss, enhanced energy, or discovering a newfound appreciation for wholesome and delicious foods.

B. Before-and-after transformations

1. Blood Pressure Improvement:
   - **Before:** High blood pressure readings and reliance on medication.
   - **After:** Normalized blood pressure levels, reduced medication dosage, and improved overall cardiovascular health.

2. Weight Loss Success:
   - **Before:** Struggled with excess weight and unhealthy eating habits.
   - **After:** Achieved significant weight loss, developed a sustainable approach to eating, and experienced increased energy levels.

3. Energy and Vitality Boost:
   - **Before:** Constant fatigue and low energy levels.
   - **After:** Increased vitality, improved focus, and a more active lifestyle.

4. Culinary Transformation:
   - **Before:** Limited cooking skills and reliance on processed foods.

- **After:** Culinary exploration, mastery of DASH-friendly recipes, and a newfound appreciation for fresh, whole ingredients.

5. Family Health Makeover:
  - **Before:** Unhealthy eating patterns affecting the entire family.
  - **After:** Shared commitment to the DASH diet, improved family health, and positive lifestyle changes for everyone.

6. Stress Management Journey:
  - **Before:** High-stress levels impacting mental well-being.
  - **After:** Implemented stress management techniques, experienced greater emotional balance, and overall improved mental health.

7. Physical Fitness Progress:
  - **Before:** Sedentary lifestyle and lack of regular exercise.
  - **After:** Increased physical activity, improved fitness levels, and a more active and enjoyable lifestyle.

8. Heart Health Transformation:
  - **Before:** Concerns about a family history of heart disease.
  - **After:** Improved cardiovascular health markers, reduced risk factors, and a proactive approach to heart well-being.

These before-and-after transformations showcase the positive impact of adopting the DASH diet, not only on physical health but also on overall well-being and lifestyle.

C. Inspirational stories to motivate beginners

1. Samantha's Journey to Heart Health:
   - Samantha embraced the DASH diet after a family history of heart disease. Through dedication and healthier choices, her blood pressure normalized, and she became a living testament to the power of lifestyle changes in promoting heart health.

2. Mark's Weight Loss Triumph:
   - Mark struggled with excess weight and low energy. With the DASH diet, he not only shed pounds but discovered a newfound love for nutritious foods. His transformation inspired others to embark on their own weight loss journeys.

3. The Smith Family's Lifestyle Makeover:
   - The Smiths, a family of four, adopted the DASH diet together. Not only did they experience improvements in their health, but the shared commitment also strengthened their bond, making healthy living a fun and inclusive family affair.

4. Jennifer's Culinary Adventure:

- Jennifer, a self-professed non-cook, transformed her relationship with food through the DASH diet. She explored diverse recipes, mastered the art of cooking, and found joy in preparing delicious and nutritious meals, proving that anyone can become a culinary enthusiast.

5. David's Stress-Free Success:

- David managed to overcome chronic stress through a combination of stress management techniques and DASH principles. His story serves as a reminder that adopting a heart-healthy lifestyle goes beyond just diet—it's about holistic well-being.

6. Emma's Fitness Evolution:

- Emma, a beginner in fitness, gradually incorporated exercise into her routine alongside the DASH diet. Her journey from a sedentary lifestyle to an active one inspires others to start small and build up, proving that every step counts on the path to well-being.

7. John's Journey from Processed to Whole Foods:

- John, once reliant on processed foods, transformed his diet with whole, nutrient-dense foods. His story motivates beginners to take small steps toward cleaner eating, emphasizing that sustainable changes yield long-lasting results.

8. Hannah's Balanced Lifestyle:

- Hannah's commitment to the DASH diet not only improved her health but also fostered a balanced lifestyle. Her story inspires others to view health as a holistic journey, where both physical and mental well-being are equally important.

These inspirational stories showcase the transformative power of adopting the DASH diet, proving that small, consistent changes can lead to significant improvements in health and overall well-being.

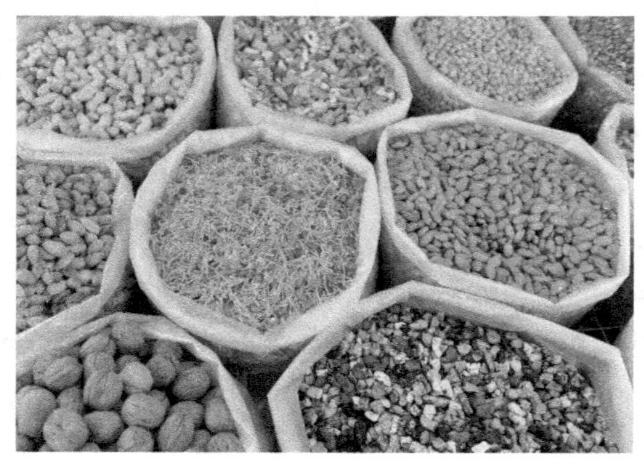

Chapter Seven

Frequently Asked Questions

1. What does DASH stand for?
   - DASH stands for Dietary Approaches to Stop Hypertension.

2. What are the main principles of the DASH diet?
   - The DASH diet emphasizes consuming a variety of nutrient-rich foods, particularly fruits, vegetables, whole grains, lean proteins, and low-fat dairy. It also recommends limiting sodium intake.

3. Is the DASH diet suitable for weight loss?
   - Yes, the DASH diet can support weight loss due to its focus on whole, nutrient-dense foods and portion control. It is often recommended for those looking to manage both blood pressure and weight.

4. Can I personalize the DASH diet to accommodate dietary restrictions?
   - Absolutely. The DASH diet is flexible and can be adapted to various dietary needs, including gluten-free, vegetarian, or vegan preferences.

5. How quickly can I expect to see results with the DASH diet?
   - Results vary, but many individuals notice improvements in blood pressure within a few weeks

of adopting the DASH diet. Changes in weight and overall well-being may take longer and depend on individual factors.

6. Are there specific recipes available for the DASH diet?
   - Yes, there are numerous DASH-friendly recipes available, ranging from breakfast options to main courses and snacks. Many cookbooks, websites, and apps provide a wealth of ideas.

7. Can I eat out while following the DASH diet?
   - Yes, you can eat out while following the DASH diet. Look for restaurants that offer whole, minimally processed foods, and ask for modifications like reducing salt in your order.

8. Is the DASH diet suitable for all age groups?
   - Yes, the DASH diet is suitable for individuals of all ages, from children to seniors. It promotes overall health and can be adapted to meet the nutritional needs of different life stages.

9. How can I manage sodium intake on the DASH diet?
   - Manage sodium intake by choosing fresh, whole foods, and minimizing processed and packaged items. Use herbs, spices, and other flavorings to season food instead of relying on salt.

10. Can I follow the DASH diet if I have diabetes?

- Yes, the DASH diet can be adapted for individuals with diabetes. It aligns with many diabetes-friendly principles, emphasizing whole foods and balanced meals.

These FAQs provide general information about the DASH diet, but individuals with specific health concerns should consult with healthcare professionals or registered dietitians for personalized advice.

A. Addressing common queries about the DASH diet

1. Is the DASH diet suitable for vegetarians or vegans?
- Yes, the DASH diet can be adapted for vegetarians or vegans by incorporating plant-based protein sources like beans, lentils, tofu, and nuts.

2. How does the DASH diet help with weight loss?
- The DASH diet aids weight loss by promoting a balanced and nutrient-dense eating pattern, which can lead to reduced calorie intake. It also encourages the consumption of whole, unprocessed foods that contribute to satiety.

3. Can I follow the DASH diet if I have gluten intolerance?
- Absolutely. The DASH diet can be modified to be gluten-free by choosing gluten-free grains like

quinoa, rice, and oats and avoiding
gluten-containing products.

4. What role does sodium play in the DASH diet,
and how can I reduce it?
   - Sodium reduction is a key aspect of the DASH
diet. To reduce sodium intake, focus on choosing
fresh, whole foods, and limit the use of processed
and packaged items. Use herbs, spices, and other
flavorings to season food instead of salt.

5. Can I eat out while following the DASH diet?
   - Yes, you can eat out on the DASH diet. Choose
restaurants that offer whole, minimally processed
foods. Ask for modifications such as reducing salt
in your order, and opt for dishes rich in fruits,
vegetables, and lean proteins.

6. Is the DASH diet only for individuals with high
blood pressure?
   - While initially designed to help manage blood
pressure, the DASH diet offers a well-rounded and
heart-healthy approach suitable for anyone looking
to improve their overall well-being, including weight
management and cardiovascular health.

7. How quickly can I expect to see changes in
blood pressure on the DASH diet?
   - Individual responses vary, but many people
notice improvements in blood pressure within a few
weeks of consistently following the DASH diet.

8. Can I consume alcohol on the DASH diet?

   - Moderate alcohol consumption is allowed on the DASH diet. However, it's essential to be mindful of portion sizes and choose drinks with lower alcohol content. It's advised to consult with a healthcare professional, especially if there are existing health conditions.

9. Is the DASH diet suitable for children?

   - Yes, the DASH diet can be adapted for children by including a variety of nutrient-dense foods suitable for their age and energy requirements. Encouraging healthy eating habits from a young age sets a foundation for lifelong well-being.

10. What are some quick and easy DASH-friendly snacks?

   - Quick DASH-friendly snacks include Greek yogurt with berries, raw vegetables with hummus, a handful of nuts, or whole fruit. These options provide a mix of nutrients without excessive sodium or added sugars.

Addressing these common queries helps individuals better understand the DASH diet and its adaptability to various dietary needs and preferences.

1. Misconception: The DASH diet is only for people with high blood pressure.

  - **Clarification:** While originally developed to manage blood pressure, the DASH diet is beneficial for anyone seeking a heart-healthy lifestyle. Its principles align with overall well-being, including weight management and cardiovascular health.

2. Misconception: The DASH diet is restrictive and lacks variety.

  - **Clarification:** The DASH diet promotes a diverse and balanced eating pattern, encouraging the consumption of various fruits, vegetables, whole grains, lean proteins, and dairy. It allows for creativity in meal planning and offers a wide range of flavorful options.

3. Misconception: Following the DASH diet requires expensive or hard-to-find ingredients.

  - **Clarification:** The DASH diet focuses on accessible, whole foods that are often affordable and readily available. It doesn't necessitate expensive specialty items, making it practical for individuals on different budgets.

4. Misconception: The DASH diet is a short-term solution.

- **Clarification:** The DASH diet is designed as a long-term, sustainable lifestyle. Its emphasis on balanced nutrition and healthy habits encourages lasting changes rather than quick fixes, promoting overall health.

5. Misconception: The DASH diet is not suitable for vegetarians or vegans.

- **Clarification:** The DASH diet is adaptable for vegetarians or vegans, emphasizing plant-based proteins like legumes and tofu. It can be customized to meet various dietary preferences while maintaining its core principles.

6. Misconception: Salt elimination is necessary on the DASH diet.

- **Clarification:** The DASH diet recommends reducing sodium intake, not eliminating it entirely. The focus is on choosing whole foods and using herbs and spices for flavor, promoting a gradual and sustainable approach to lower sodium intake.

7. Misconception: The DASH diet is not effective for weight loss.

- **Clarification:** The DASH diet supports weight loss by promoting whole, nutrient-dense foods and portion control. Numerous studies have shown its effectiveness in both improving cardiovascular health and aiding weight management.

8. Misconception: The DASH diet is too time-consuming to follow.

- **Clarification:** The DASH diet accommodates various lifestyles, and many recipes are quick and easy to prepare. Batch cooking and meal planning can further streamline the process, making it feasible for individuals with busy schedules.

9. Misconception: Alcohol is not allowed on the DASH diet.

- **Clarification:** Moderate alcohol consumption is permitted on the DASH diet. However, it's essential to be mindful of portion sizes, choose lower-alcohol beverages, and consider individual health conditions.

10. Misconception: Results on the DASH diet are not backed by scientific evidence.

- **Clarification:** The DASH diet is extensively supported by scientific research, demonstrating its effectiveness in reducing blood pressure, improving overall cardiovascular health, and aiding in weight management.

Addressing these misconceptions with evidence-based information helps individuals make informed decisions about adopting the DASH diet, fostering a better understanding of its principles and benefits.

Conclusion

In conclusion, the DASH diet, or Dietary Approaches to Stop Hypertension, offers a comprehensive and evidence-based approach to promoting heart health and overall well-being. From its roots in managing blood pressure to its broader applications in weight management, the DASH diet stands out as a sustainable lifestyle choice. Its core principles encourage the consumption of nutrient-dense foods, emphasizing a diverse range of fruits, vegetables, whole grains, lean proteins, and low-fat dairy.

Through the journey of exploring the DASH diet, beginners can uncover not only a path to improved cardiovascular health but also a transformative lifestyle. The emphasis on flexibility, adaptability to different dietary preferences, and the integration of stress management and exercise make the DASH diet a holistic approach to well-being.

From understanding the basics of the DASH diet and its principles to debunking common misconceptions, this journey encompasses valuable insights into creating a sustainable, heart-healthy lifestyle. The real-life experiences, success stories, and inspirational transformations underscore the positive impact that adopting the DASH diet can have on individuals of various backgrounds and ages.

As beginners embark on their DASH diet journey, armed with knowledge about meal planning, stress management, exercise integration, and personalized adaptations, they can confidently stride toward a healthier and more balanced lifestyle. The DASH diet is not merely a set of dietary guidelines; it is an invitation to explore a world of flavorful and nutritious foods while nurturing overall well-being.

In this conclusion, let it be a reminder that the DASH diet is not a restrictive regimen but a sustainable and enjoyable way of living that promotes lasting health benefits. As individuals commit to this heart-healthy journey, they pave the way for a future marked by vitality, balance, and a steadfast commitment to well-being.

A. Recap of key DASH principles

1. Emphasize Whole Foods:
   - Prioritize whole, minimally processed foods, such as fruits, vegetables, whole grains, lean proteins, and low-fat dairy.

2. Balanced Nutrient Intake:
   - Strive for a balanced distribution of macronutrients, including carbohydrates, proteins, and healthy fats, to support overall well-being.

3. Limit Sodium Intake:

- Reduce sodium intake by choosing fresh foods and using herbs, spices, and other flavorings to season meals, promoting heart health.

4. Portion Control:
   - Be mindful of portion sizes to avoid overeating and promote weight management, an integral part of the DASH diet's success.

5. Adaptability to Preferences:
   - Tailor the DASH diet to individual preferences, accommodating dietary needs such as vegetarian, vegan, or gluten-free preferences.

6. Stress Management:
   - Recognize the impact of stress on health and incorporate stress management techniques, such as mindfulness and relaxation, into the lifestyle.

7. Regular Physical Activity:
   - Integrate regular exercise into the routine for overall cardiovascular health and well-being, aligning with the DASH diet's holistic approach.

8. Flexibility and Long-Term Commitment:
   - View the DASH diet as a flexible, long-term commitment, allowing for occasional indulgences while maintaining a consistent focus on heart-healthy choices.

9. Community Support:

- Seek support from communities or social networks with similar health goals, fostering encouragement, shared experiences, and motivation.

10. Holistic Lifestyle Integration:
   - Integrate DASH principles into various aspects of daily life, including stress management, physical activity, and social connections, creating a holistic approach to well-being.

By revisiting and incorporating these key DASH principles, individuals can confidently navigate their journey toward a heart-healthy lifestyle, enjoying the benefits of improved cardiovascular health and overall well-being.

B. Encouragement for beginners on their journey to better health

Congratulations on taking this important step toward prioritizing your well-being! Embracing the DASH diet is a meaningful choice that lays the foundation for a healthier, more vibrant life. As you begin this journey, here's some encouragement to guide you:

1. Celebrate Small Wins:
   - Acknowledge and celebrate every small achievement along the way. Whether it's choosing a nutritious snack or incorporating an extra serving

of vegetables, each step contributes to your overall success.

2. Embrace Flexibility:
 - Understand that adopting a new lifestyle takes time. Embrace flexibility in your approach, allowing yourself the freedom to enjoy occasional treats while staying committed to the principles of the DASH diet.

3. Listen to Your Body:
 - Pay attention to how your body responds to the changes. Notice the positive shifts in energy, mood, and overall well-being. This awareness will strengthen your connection with your body and its needs.

4. Enjoy the Culinary Adventure:
 - Explore the world of delicious and nutritious foods that the DASH diet offers. Get creative in the kitchen, try new recipes, and savor the diverse flavors of whole, unprocessed ingredients.

5. Build a Support System:
 - Share your journey with friends, family, or join online communities. Having a support system can provide encouragement, motivation, and a sense of camaraderie as you navigate the challenges and successes together.

6. Patience is Key:

- Transformations take time. Be patient with yourself as you adapt to new habits and make sustainable changes. The journey is as important as the destination.

7. Prioritize Self-Care:
   - Beyond diet and exercise, prioritize self-care. Take moments for relaxation, indulge in activities you enjoy, and ensure you're nurturing both your physical and mental well-being.

8. Believe in Your Potential:
   - You have the power to shape your health and future. Believe in your potential to make positive, lasting changes. Every effort you put in contributes to a healthier and happier you.

Remember, this journey is about progress, not perfection. Each day is a new opportunity to make choices that align with your health goals. Stay committed, stay positive, and cherish the journey toward a healthier, more vibrant version of yourself. You've got this!

C. Final thoughts on sustaining a DASH-friendly lifestyle.

In sustaining a DASH-friendly lifestyle, it's essential to view it not as a temporary endeavor but as a lifelong commitment to your well-being. Here are some final thoughts to guide you on this journey:

1. Consistency Over Perfection:
   - Strive for consistency rather than perfection. Small, steady changes are more sustainable and can lead to long-term success. Focus on making the DASH principles a natural part of your daily routine.

2. Adaptability is Key:
   - Life is dynamic, and your approach to a healthy lifestyle should be too. Be adaptable to changes, and find ways to incorporate DASH principles into various situations, from social events to travel.

3. Reflect and Learn:
   - Regularly reflect on your progress and learn from your experiences. What worked well? What challenges did you overcome? Continuous self-reflection empowers you to make informed choices on your journey.

4. Supportive Networks:
   - Cultivate a supportive network. Share your goals with friends or family, join communities with similar health aspirations, and lean on your support system during both triumphs and challenges.

5. Holistic Health Focus:
   - Recognize that health goes beyond just what you eat. Prioritize stress management, adequate sleep, and regular physical activity. A holistic approach ensures comprehensive well-being.

6. Set Realistic Goals:

   - Set achievable and realistic goals. Break down larger objectives into smaller, manageable steps. Celebrate each milestone along the way, fostering motivation and a positive mindset.

7. Enjoy the Journey:

   - Embrace the joy of discovering new foods, flavors, and a healthier way of living. The DASH-friendly lifestyle is not a restrictive path; it's an invitation to savor the richness of life with well-balanced choices.

8. Self-Compassion:

   - Be kind to yourself. Understand that everyone faces setbacks, and it's okay. Approach challenges with self-compassion, learn from them, and continue moving forward on your journey.

By integrating these principles into your lifestyle, the DASH-friendly approach becomes not just a diet but a fulfilling and sustainable way of living. As you navigate each day with mindfulness, adaptability, and a commitment to your well-being, you'll find that sustaining a DASH-friendly lifestyle becomes a natural and rewarding part of your life's journey. Here's to a future filled with health, vitality, and a heart-healthy lifestyle!